Your Shadow on the
FLOOR

Your Shadow on the
FLOOR

A Survivor's Guide to Investing

James William Schwarz

To order additional copies of this book, contact:
Xlibris Corporation
1-888-795-4274
www.Xlibris.com
Orders@Xlibris.com
118580

Contents

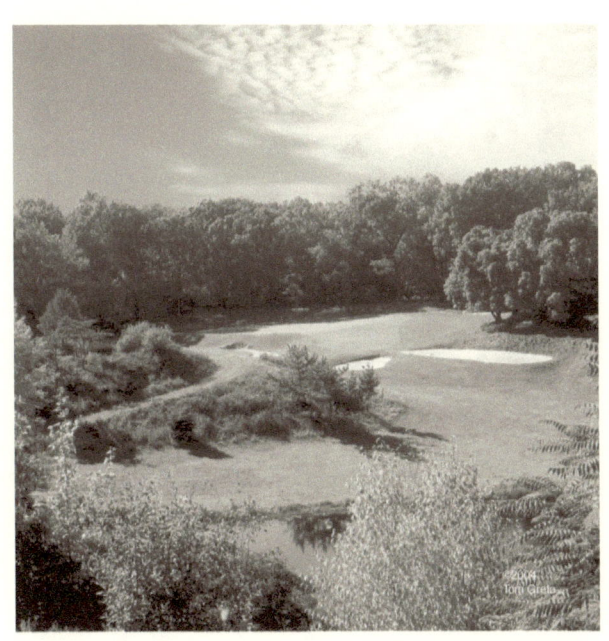

Dedicated to my father and mother,
John Joseph Schwarz and Nancy.
You put me on the right path, Pop.
You gave me life.
Thank you.

"Happiness = Beauty + enough" (Aristotle).

Being able to pay your bills is large.

Discover your risk appetite / risk aversion and your significant others.

Successful investment is making money in good times and bad.

Taxes will be your biggest financial burden.

Laughter is the best medicine.

Let me start with a few words about where I am coming from.

I was a paperboy, busboy, technician for a hospital, taxi driver, counselor, retail clerk, and more. I worked very hard through school and was lucky to get a professional job as a computer programmer, sometimes working two full-time jobs as I attended to my studies. I paid for 90 percent of my education and loans, and I can look the world in the eye.

I was fortunate to get a great education where I learned to handle money, and I graduated from college with four dollars and a job.

I survived the corporate world, cancer, a brain tumor, and I am battling MS (multiple sclerosis). "You play it as it lies," in the words of golf's great Bobby Jones. One day at a time. My wife was laid off, however, after twenty-five years of hard work. An e-mail to say good luck?

I was not happy.

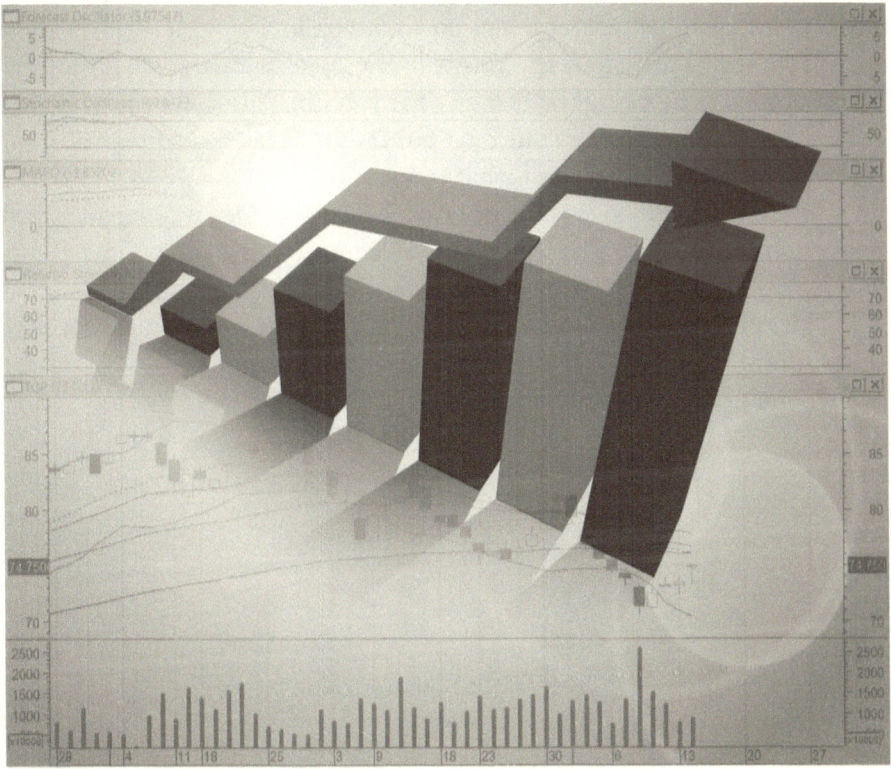

It is not a condemnation of the system. This is life, and it is not fair. The sooner you get it, the better.

This is how to fight back. You may have become ill by fate or *service to your country.*

There is hope and enjoyment derived from investing.

This is a guide for young and old confronting the difficult task of managing their investment needs in a confusing and sometimes treacherous environment. This is a whole life, holistic approach to investing for the long run.

As the title says, today more than ever, sometimes the only thing behind you is *your shadow on the floor.*

The good news is, this is the time to take responsibility and become empowered to build your future safely, slowly, and consistently.

Additionally, if you become self-sufficient, you can take an employment route that you will love and not depend on a company for your needs. You may choose a path that is less conventional but personally rewarding. Suppose you find that you are the best widget maker and you love making widgets. You will be happier if you do what you love.

Happiness is a huge asset. You will also reap comparative advantage, which is created by being the best at what you do. This is not meant to say that you should go out on your own but rather to take advantage of what is offered as far as benefits and what to look for.

I am not going to give you stock tips. The whole idea is to learn to find opportunities yourself. The most valuable commodity is *time.* Time allows you to make mistakes, repair your mistakes, and build wealth.

Older people like me often wonder where it went. You blink and you're thirty. Blink again and you are forty, and so on. The good news is that the sooner you begin, the easier it gets.

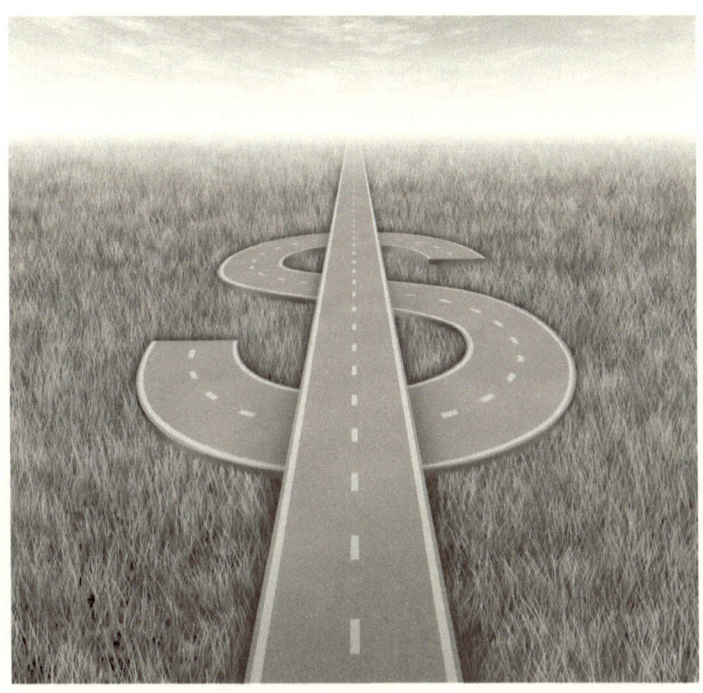

Let me introduce again to two words: *compounded interest.*

Compound interest arises when interest is added to the principal, so that, from that moment on, the interest that has been added also earns interest. This addition of interest to the principal is called *compounding.* A bank account, for example, may have its interest compounded every year: in this case, an account with ¤1000 initial principal and 20% interest per year would have a balance of ¤1200 at the end of the first year, ¤1440 at the end of the second year, and so on.

In order to define an interest rate fully, and enable one to compare it with other interest rates, the interest rate *and* the compounding frequency must be disclosed. Since most people prefer to think of rates as a yearly percentage, many governments require financial institutions to disclose the equivalent yearly compounded interest rate on deposits or advances. For instance, the yearly rate for a loan with 1% interest per month is approximately 12.68% per annum ($1.01^{12} - 1$). This equivalent yearly rate may be referred to as annual percentage rate (APR), annual equivalent rate (AER), annual percentage yield, effective interest rate, *effective annual rate,* and by other terms. When a fee is charged up front to obtain a loan, APR usually counts that cost as well as the compound interest in converting to the equivalent rate. These government requirements assist consumers to compare the actual costs of borrowing more easily. For any given interest rate and compounding frequency, an "equivalent" rate for any different compounding frequency exists.

Compound interest may be contrasted with simple interest, where interest is not added to the principal (there is no compounding). Compound interest is standard in finance and economics, and simple interest is used infrequently (although certain financial products may contain elements of simple interest).

I was fortunate to have a parent who was investing literate. My father bestowed on my siblings and me at an early age the benefits of investing for the long run. He did not do the investing for us but rather gave us the information of the benefit of time. He said that money can grow like an amoeba, which replicates by splitting and becomes a new life. So is the concept of money wisely invested.

Risk (Most to Least)

- Non US common stock
- Non US corporate bonds
- US stocks
- Preferred stocks
- US corporate bonds
- Municipal bonds
- Treasury bonds
- US bills and notes

Eventually, the average cost per share of the security will become smaller and smaller. Dollar-cost averaging lessens the risk of investing a large amount in a single investment at the wrong time. For example, you decide to purchase $100 worth of XYZ each month for three months. In January, XYZ is worth $33, so you buy three shares. In February, XYZ is worth $25, so you buy four additional shares this time. Finally, in March, XYZ is worth $20, so you buy five shares. In total, you purchased 12 shares for an average price of approximately $25 each. In the UK, it is known as "pound-cost averaging." Read more at *http://www.investopedia. com/terms/d/dollarcostaveraging. asp#ixzz1ygCDOGSD*

YOUR ACCOUNTS

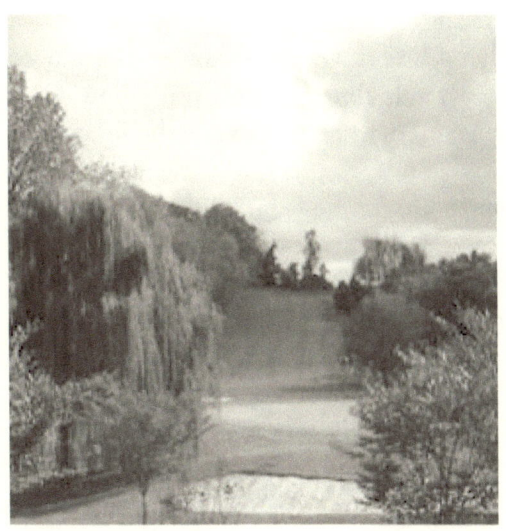

T HE TOTAL OF your wealth is not just the bottom line of your accounts. It is the sum total of all your investments, including company benefits, real estate, your hobbies, your health and life insurance, and more.

In the hierarchy, your base should be built on a pyramid where the foundation is rock solid for the long run, and as you climb the pyramid, you can take more risk but safely.

Diversification in bonds and stocks because they move inversely to each other is wise.

Your bond exposure is suggested to match the percentage of your age. For example, if you are twenty-five, you should have 25 percent in bond funds. Each January, I rebalance the portfolio 1 percent.

I do not invest in single company bond but rather long—, intermediate—, and short-term bond mutual funds. Part of your portfolio should be in gold or gold miners because gold acts inversely to the dollar. Physical metal bullion should be accumulated at the right price and time.

Bonds and bond funds are negatively affected by inflation and interest rates. As interest rates go up, long-term bond goes down because newly issued bonds have better yields. The smart play is a diversified portfolio of short—, intermediate—, and long-term bonds.

Everyone needs to discover their style. My style evolved over thirty years of investing. I have witnessed many recessions and downturns and was fortunate to survive them intact and employed. There is no optimum style, but there are suggestions.

My style is that a little investment now can produce an above average rate of return in a variable time period if you follow the suggestions.

When choosing an investment I follow the following:

First suggestion: Do not buy crap, like garbage in, garbage out. If you buy crap, it will produce crap

Second suggestion: Not all experts have your interests in mind, so do not believe what you read. I was amazed to find out that some people's job is and was solely to inflate the daily volume, hence making an equity move and selling into the rally.

Third suggestion: Your opinion and view of reality is just as keen as the opinion of an MBA from the Wharton School. Peter Lynch, the great investment manager, would watch what his children were buying to make investment decisions with great success.

Fourth suggestion: There is no get-rich-quick formula.

Humor Break
Irish Golfer

A golfer playing in Ireland hooked his drive into the woods. Looking for his ball, he finds a little leprechaun flat on his back, a big bump on his head, and the golfer's ball beside him. Horrified, the golfer gets his water bottle from the cart and poured it over the little guy, reviving him.

"Arrgh! What happened?" the leprechaun asks.

"I'm afraid I hit you with my golf ball," the golfer says.

"Oh, I see. Well, ye got me fair and square? Ye get three wishes, so whaddya want?"

"Thank God, you're all right!" the golfer answers in relief. "I don't want anything, I'm just glad you're OK, and I apologize." And the golfer walks off.

"What a nice guy," the leprechaun says to himself. I have to do something for him. I'll give him the three things I would want—a great golf game, all the money he ever needs, and a fantastic sex life."

A year goes by and the golfer is back. On the same hole, he again hits a bad drive into the woods, and the leprechaun is there waiting for him.

"'Twas me that made ye hit the ball here," the little guy says. "I just want to ask ye, how's yer golf game?"

"My game is fantastic!" the golfer answers. "I'm an internationally famous golfer now." He adds, "By the way, it's good to see you're all right."

"Oh, I'm fine now, thank ye. I did that fer yer golf game, you know. And tell me, how's yer money situation?"

"Why, it's just wonderful!" the golfer states. "When I need cash, I just reach in my pocket and pull out one-hundred-dollar bills I didn't even know were there!"

"I did that fer ye also. And tell me, how's yer sex life?"

The golfer blushes, turns his head away in embarrassment, and says shyly, "It's OK."

"C'mon, c'mon now," urges the leprechaun, "I'm wanting to know if I did a good job. How many times a week?"

Blushing even more, the golfer looks around then whispers, "Once, sometimes twice a week."

"What?" responds the leprechaun in shock. "That's all? Only once or twice a week?"

"Well," says the golfer, "I figure that's not bad for a Catholic priest in a small parish."

YOUR EDUCATION

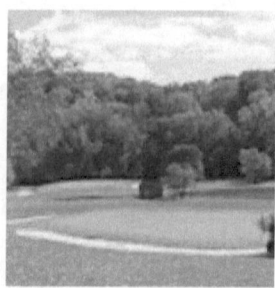

YOUR EDUCATION, WHETHER it is a trade or traditional education, is a huge asset that must be nourished over your lifetime. It is important to become a lifelong learner. Change is constant, and new technologies are always being invented. Education is something that cannot be taken away when achieved honestly. It is status, and the benefits continue.

What I found is that a general education combined with a focused trade is a powerful combination. Concentrate on what is needed every day and by all so that the downturns do not affect you. General education requirements are the same for all colleges. It is not where you start but rather where you end up.

My problem is the debt incurred by the student. One acquaintance owes $125,000. The cost of an education far surpasses inflation. I would recommend starting at a reasonable school and finish at the prestigious institution.

YOUR AVOCATIONS

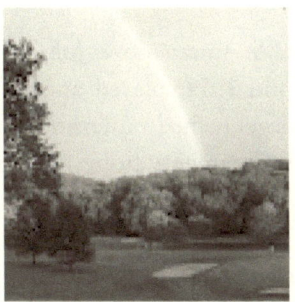

YOUR HOBBIES AND avocations are very important for maintaining your health and mental balance. Also, these activities can be a source of lifetime friendships.

My father golfed and I golfed, and it became a source of communication during my teens, when it was sometimes difficult to find common ground and bridging the generation gap. It can be an expensive hobby both in terms of time and funds.

After twenty-some years working as a computer programmer, I received an invite to join a country club sponsored through a longtime member named Joe Boyle from Havertown, who was and is the neighbor of Pat McElwee.

Edgmont Country Club is owned and run by Pam and Peter Mariani. It is our Happy Valley. I cannot say enough of the beauty of this course and the great people that work there: Al Balukas, the starter, is friendly with Ed Dougherty, who played on the tour; Jeff Herb and Craig; Frank Smiley, Mike Taylor, and Mike in the pro shop; Norm and Mike, the bartenders; Lexie, Earl, and many more.

Many great folks, including Victor Stitz who is a member and a friend. Self made and a boxer. Coming from almost poverty to wealth, Victor rose above it all. Deeply devoted to his family, he sponsors a dinner each year for the needy. More people each year anonymously with his kids helping. Pam is an author with published children's novels. I also got to meet Skee Riegel.

Robert Henry "Skee" Riegel (November 25, 1914-February 22, 2009) was an American professional golfer.

Riegel attended West Point, Hobart College, and Lafayette College where he played football and baseball but not golf. He took up golf at the age of 23.[1] During World War II, he was a flying instructor for the US Army Air Corp in Arkadelphia, Arkansas.

Riegel won the 1947 U.S. Amateur over Johnny Dawson at the Pebble Beach Golf Links, 2 and 1. He played on the Walker Cup teams of 1947 and 1949.[1] Riegel turned professional in 1950 and played in 11 straight Masters Tournaments from 1947 to 1957. In the 1951 Masters Tournament, he was tied with Sam Snead after three rounds and finished second to Ben Hogan by two strokes. Riegel finished second to Ted Kroll in the 1952 Insurance City Open.

Riegel stopped playing full time in 1952-1953. He served as head pro at Radnor Valley Country Club from 1954 to 1961 and then became involved in the ownership of York Road Country Club in Bucks County, Pennsylvania.[1]

Riegel was the Pro Emeritus at the Cape May National Golf Club in Cape May, New Jersey. He was often found walking the grounds with his poodle John Paul. Cape May National holds a large amount of history, with a number of articles about "Skee" on the walls of its Clubhouse, as well a number of plaques located on the 18th tee.

There is also a stone remembrance at Edgmont. Also, the first tournament of the year is named for Shag Crawford. Shag passed on as well and his son umpired in the MLB (Major League Baseball). I met him once during the tournament.

Henry Charles "Shag" Crawford (August 30, 1916–July 11, 2007)[1] [2] was an American umpire in Major League Baseball who worked in the National League from 1956 to 1975.[3] During his twenty seasons in the National League, Crawford worked more than 3,100 games and as a home plate umpire was notable for getting in a low crouch and resting his hands on the back of the catcher in front of him. Crawford wore number 2 after the National League adopted numbers for its umpires, which was then transferred to his son Jerry Crawford, who wore it from 1976 until his 2010 retirement.

Crawford was born in Philadelphia, Pennsylvania. Growing up, he played baseball and football and was involved in boxing, and later played in the minor leagues as a catcher in the Philadelphia Phillies' system.[4] He served in the United States Navy during World War II, and was on the destroyer Walke when its bridge was struck by a Japanese kamikaze on January 6, 1945 during the invasion of Luzon, in which commanding officer George Fleming Davis suffered fatal injuries and was awarded the Medal of Honor. Crawford became a minor league umpire in 1950, working for two months in the Canadian-American League before moving to the Eastern League from 1951 to 1953 and the American Association in from 1954 to 1955; his contract was purchased by the National League in November 1955.

During his career, he officiated three World Series (1961, 1963, 1969), ejecting Baltimore manager Earl Weaver in Game 4 of the 1969 Series for arguing balls and strikes, the first managerial ejection in World Series competition since 1935, two National League Championship Series (1971, 1974), and All-Star Games in 1959 (first game), 1961 (first game) and 1968; he worked behind the plate for the 1968 All-Star Game.[1] On June 4, 1964, he was the third base umpire for Sandy Koufax's third no-hitter. Crawford was relieved of his duties in 1975 for refusing to work the World Series that year, due to a rotational system implemented for selection of World Series umpires, over the traditional assignment by merit.

Crawford married Vivian Gallagher on November 2, 1940, and they had three sons and a daughter, residing in Haverford, Pennsylvania; two of their sons, Jerry and Joey, also became sports officials. Jerry was a National League umpire from 1976 until 2010, and Joey has been a National Basketball Association referee since 1977. Shag Crawford worked the first game at Philadelphia's Veterans Stadium in 1971 and stood with Jerry at home plate when the lineup cards were presented before the final game at the ballpark in 2003.

Fair, fun, and friendly and historic.

Pat McElwee, who joined with me, has been my friend through "sick and sin" since we were students at Cardinal O'Hara in the early '70s. Along with Joe, I was cosponsored by the inimitable Teddy Vanderslice, whom I befriended while coaching through Larchmont Little League in Marple Township. I did not know that he worked at the Philadelphia Inquirer with Pat as a premier salesman who could sell the devil his own soul.

Ted is one of those unforgettable, larger-than-life people that you meet in life, tall and rounder with skinny legs like Babe Ruth. A former baseball player at Monsignor Bonner (a perennial rival for O'Hara), he had a wit that few could match.

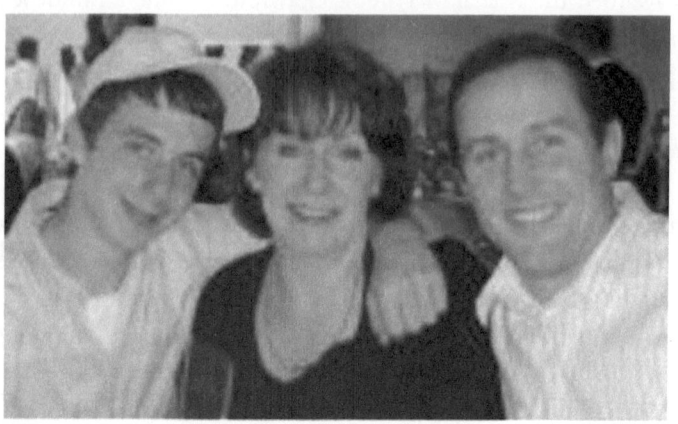

One summer day not too long ago, we were playing the eighteenth hole. I was driving Ted to his ball in the center of the fairway, not long but enough to have a clean shot in to the green. On this dogleg left, Ted walked over to his ball and prepared to swing, when about three hundred or so multicolored butterflies engulfed him where he stood.

As quickly as they came they disappeared. He fired his shot on the green in two.

Magic.

He never said a word.

We played for years before with the guild from the *Inquirer* on an annual pilgrimage to Ocean City, Maryland, and later Atlantic City. Ted would get numerous strangers shaking his hand because of his resemblance to Eagles coach Andy Reid, which he would not deny, which would give us status among the other golfers on holiday.

Carl and Carl Jr., Bill, Dave, Mike, Obie and Eddie Curtin (who recently died unexpectedly). Daily matches and points. Great fun.

Pat was telling Teddy one day about Maureen's (Pat's wife) habit of shopping at the same time each Saturday. Pat said that she was out the door each weekend at ten with a huge smile and determination. Explaining this to Ted, he said that he thought there was some funny business going on.

Pat said he thought she was having an affair. Ted looked Pat directly in the eye and said, "Ten o'clock . . . I think she's cheating on me too!"

Didn't sit well with Pat, but I thought it funny. Ted does not have the discretion gene.

Later still, Ted told me in confidence that he needed a kidney transplant. I was worried. Because of his diabetes, his kidneys were failing. I kept his confidence, and when he could not play on really hot days, the pros and staff at Edgmont asked me what was going on. I did my best and explained that Ted had a condition.

Without hesitation together they all said at once, "What is it? Mental?"

His wife, Terry, gave him one of her kidneys. A 1 percent chance that beat the odds. Three years and counting. Miracles do occur every day.

One of my most memorable experiences was a day playing by myself on the back nine at course named Cobbs Creek. I was on the tee of the seventeenth par three when a twosome was cutting through and asked to join up with me. A white guy and a solid-looking black man approached and we shook hands. The black man looked familiar, and when he extended his hand and shook mine, I was impressed by his long spongy fingers and firm grip.

I remarked that he looked like Irv Cross, the former Philadelphia Eagle and sports analyst for CBS. I said he was the spitting image of Irv Cross, a.k.a. Sir Paperhead, a name given to him in his playing days for his propensity for concussions.

"I am Irv Cross," he responded in his classic CBS television voice.

I never met anyone on TV or a pro football player.

We proceeded to play the seventeenth, which is a medium par three over a deep gully with a sloping green back to front. I don't remember how well we played the hole or the results, but I was excited to play with them.

We walked together up the hill through the trees to the eighteenth. They were watering the tee with those circular sprinklers that, when placed with a club in the middle of the works, would stop the revolution and spray sideways in a V, which gave you a path to hit without getting wet.

The partner of Irv proceeded to place a club in the first of two sprinklers closest to us setting up the first V. I walked to the second to do the same to the second.

With my bag still on my shoulder, I took out a club to place in the sprinkler and bent down and proceeded to spill all my clubs on the tee without stopping the water from the revolving sprinkler, thoroughly soaking me and all my clubs. I looked back in embarrassment at Irv and his partner, who were now kindly laughing, trying not to be too visible with their laughter.

When I achieved my objective and picked my soaking clubs and dripping self, I deposited the clubs in my bag, and all Irv said was that, that was one of the funniest things he had ever seen.

We played the eighteenth together and shook hands with smiles at the end, and they wished me luck.

True story.

Get involved. Shop around. Do what you love, whatever it is. Join groups to maintain the connections with others of equal interests.

YOUR HEALTH

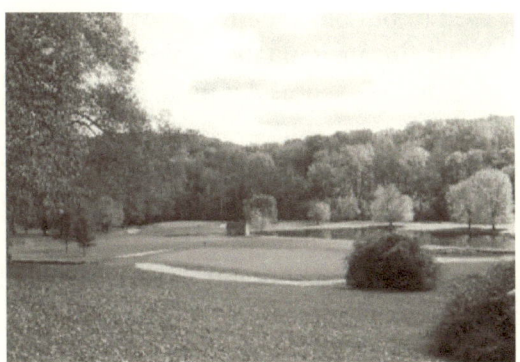

YOUR HEALTH IS the most important. Without it you are at a loss. I was cruising along when I was felled by illness.

Nothing I could do. No cure.

So is life.

No cure yet.

Use a broker to get the best deal. They do not charge you and can save you significant premium.

You can find one on the internet.

Humor Break

At dawn the telephone rings. "Hello, Senor Rod? This is Ernesto, you know, the caretaker at your country house."

"Ah yes, Ernesto. What can I do for you? Is there a problem?"

"Um, I am just calling to advise you, Senor Rod, that your parrot, he is dead."

"My parrot? Dead? The one that won the international competition?"

"Sí, Senor, that's the one."

"Damn! That's a pity! I spent a small fortune on that bird. What did he die from?"

"From eating the rotten meat, Senor Rod."

"Rotten meat? Who the hell fed him rotten meat?"

"Nobody, Senor. He ate the meat of the dead horse."

"Dead horse? What dead horse?"

"The Thoroughbred, Senor Rod."

"My prize-winning Thoroughbred is dead?"

"Yes, Senor Rod. He died from all that work pulling the water cart."

"Are you sh—tting me? What water cart?"

"The one we used to put out the fire, Senor."

"Good Lord! What fire are you talking about, man?"

"The one at your house, Senor! A candle fell and the curtains caught on fire."

"What the hell? Are you saying that my mansion is destroyed because of a candle!"

"Yes, Senor Rod."

"But there's electricity at the house! What was the candle for?"

"For the funeral, Senor Rod."

"WHAT BLOODY FUNERAL?"

"Your wife's, Senor Rod. She showed up very late one night, and I thought she was a thief, so I hit her with your new TaylorMade SuperQuad 460 golf club."

Silence . . . Long silence . . .

"Ernesto, if you broke that driver, you're in deep sh—t!"

Lifelong health maintenance is important. Do not skip the checkups. Your teeth are an asset that must be maintained for your health and your wallet. Nothing is more expensive than dental work. If you do not maintain your teeth, you can develop illnesses like heart problems.

A good friend of mine had an employee that was dentist phobic. He developed a heart disease and died at fifty-five. A regular cleaning may prevent dentures, crowns, and other very expensive procedures, plus a nice smile always helps job interviews.

While we are discussing your teeth, one thing that my father told me rings very true. He said that everywhere you go, you will be judged by what comes out of your mouth. You will be either praised or negatively judged by your choice of words, your diction, your language, and your volume in all professional pursuits. Your treatment of service personnel will be viewed as negative if you do not treat all with respect.

Also, foulmouthed behavior is a negative, and you should treat others with respect even though you may not think that they deserve your mindfulness. This simple truth will affect you.

YOUR VICES

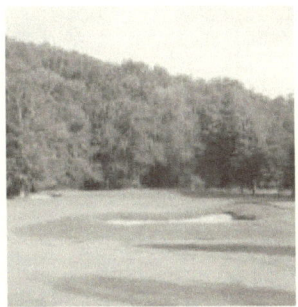

YOUR VICES WILL affect your wealth negatively more than any recession or periods of unemployment. Being immoderate with any vice will also affect your health and your relationships. A run-in with the law will cost you for legal fees and possible fines. Like I tell my youngest—fly straight or it will cost you.

Ruining your relationships will also hurt you because you need the support of your friends and they need you.

Alcohol is socially acceptable, but a DWI (driving while intoxicated) could cost plenty as far as car insurance rates, fines, or worse.

Cigarettes are very expensive and deadly. Suppose instead of smoking you invest in a closes end fund at seven dollars a share paying an eight percent dividend monthly.

One pack equals one share.

Compounded interest turns your cigarettes into an $43,870 over ten years. $133,000 over twenty and $326,000 over 30 years.

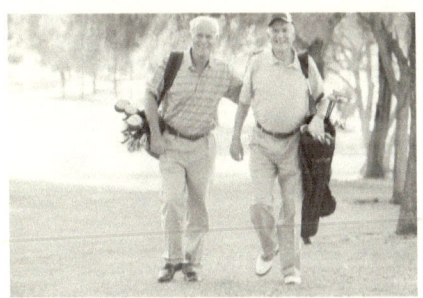

YOUR FRIENDS

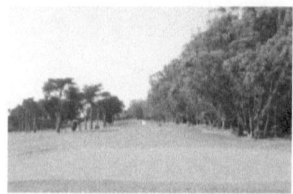

I WAS VERY FORTUNATE to have found lifetime and loyal friends: Frank Dinunzio, Tom Geddis, Pat McElwee, Ted Vanderslice, and Guy Matteo. I continue to see them although one has moved away.

We go to Myrtle Beach each year to play golf and laugh like sophomores. They motivated me to be better than I was going.

Competition breeds wealth. Friends help in hard times. Parents die. Divorce happens. Illnesses occur. Your friends will affect your future more than you know. When you find a true friend, you are blessed and never let that slip away.

A man in the Safeway Store in Texas tries to buy half a head of lettuce. The very young produce assistant tells him that they sell only whole heads of lettuce. The man persists and asks to see the manager. The boy says he'll ask his manager about it.

Walking into the back room, the boy said to his manager, "Some a—hole wants to buy half a head of lettuce." As he finished his sentence, he turned to find the man standing right behind him, so he added, "And this gentleman has kindly offered to buy the other half."

The manager approved the deal, and the man went on his way. Later the manager said to the boy, "I was impressed with the way you got yourself out of that situation earlier. We like people who think on their feet here. Where are you from, son?"

"Canada, sir," the boy replied.

"Well, why did you leave Canada?" the manager asked.

The boy said, "Sir, there's nothing but whores and hockey players up there."

"Really?" said the manager. "My wife is from Canada."

"No sh—t?" replied the boy. "Who'd she play for?"

INVESTING 101

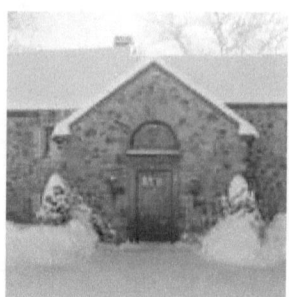

TO BEGIN YOUR investment strategy to build wealth throughout your career, take advantage of the professional money managers in mutual funds. Many companies have them as a part of a traditional IRA (individual retirement arrangement).

Vanguard is a trustee. These individuals do this for a living. Their success is their paycheck. I prefer Vanguard because they are the original and their costs are low.

There are hundreds of choices for mutual funds. There are choices that make your investments for retirement easy because they are managed over a lifetime. These are lifetime cycle mutual funds. You choose your approximate year of retirement.

Suppose that date is 2050. The professionals will manage the fund over the span and change the allocations for you into investments that reflect income-producing assets that do not have a chance of losing value as you get closer to retirement.

Generally, as you get closer to retirement, you want to be in bond-oriented funds as previous mentioned to reflect your age. These funds are generally invested in indexes. Index funds have lower costs.

Fixed income investing is A, B, C, D: *a*nnuities, *b*onds, and *c*ertificates of *d*eposits.

There are also annuity plans that provide a great degree of safety and a moderate return. We set up an annuity for the youngest and added nothing over eighteen years partly because we forgot about it. One hundred and fifty dollars turned into $2,347. I strongly suggest variable annuities for children either yours or as gifts.

Some funds have a dividend yield. Some pay yearly, quarterly, and monthly. Many pay capital gains generally at the end of the year.

Happy Holidays!

Be careful not to sell before the end of the year before capital gains are paid. Generally, bond funds pay monthly with a healthy dividend but not much of capital appreciation. When you are young, you are looking for capital appreciation. That means the price will increase but also the risk. The markets are the risk-reward paradox.

Along with risk, there is volatility. Volatility in a stock is measure by its beta. A beta over 1.0 is volatile. Volatility is sometimes good.

Mutual Fund Focus

Many choices.

Mutual funds are also divided between large and small company focus, balanced, blended, and many more. Blends divide assets between growth and value equities. Blends are less volatile and less risky than pure growth funds.

A balanced fund has bonds and stocks in its portfolio. Vanguard's Wellesley fund is a good example. It is less risky and pays a good dividend.

An area that did very well over many years is the small caps. These small companies can provide enormous gains but can get hurt in bad times.

The simple truth is, large conglomerates with foreign exposure and make many everyday products make up a large percent of mutual funds.

You have heard of the blue chips. That is Clorox, Proctor & Gamble, Johnson & Johnson, et al. They survive the storms because they have products that people need and use every day.

A group that I like is consumer non-cyclical, personal, and household products. This category includes Coke, Proctor & Gamble, Clorox, and Colgate-Palmolive. They pay a healthy dividend and are fairly recession proof.

Diversification

The USA is currently the leader, but growth is seen in emerging economies in China, Brazil, India, and Russia. Many mutual funds invest in these countries, including Europe. Growth is in emerging economies that have a growing middle class that has growing expendable income.

Company Contributions

If your company contributes a percentage to your 401K, then invest up to that amount and take advantage of the benefit. A portion when you are young should be to hold small caps because over the last fifty years, they have appreciated the most.

My view at 53

Vanguard Wellington Fund Investor Shares	0021-88026942478
Vanguard Windsor Fund Investor Shares	0022-88026942478
Vanguard Wellesley Income Fund Investor Shares	0027-88026942478
Vanguard High-Yield Corporate Fund Investor Shares	0029-88026942478
Vanguard Short-Term Investment-Grade Fund Investor Shares	0039-88026942478
Vanguard International Value Fund	0046-88026942478
Vanguard Windsor II Fund Investor Shares	0073-88026942478
Vanguard International Growth Fund Investor Shares	0081-88026942478
Vanguard Target Retirement 2025 Fund	0304-88026942478
Vanguard Target Retirement 2035 Fund	0305-88026942478
Vanguard 500 Index Fund Admiral Shares	0540-88026942478
Vanguard Small-Cap Index Fund Admiral Shares	0548-88026942478
Vanguard Long-Term Investment-Grade Fund Admiral Shares §	0568-88026942478
Vanguard Total International Stock Index Fund Admiral Shares	0569-88026942478
Vanguard Target Retirement 2020	2-88026942478

INVESTING 201

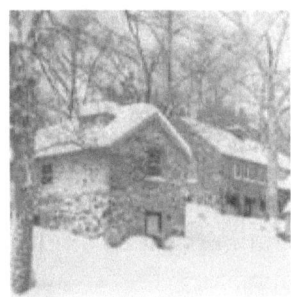

D O NOT RELY solely on your mutual fund.

This account is savings for life events, with a five—to fifteen-year window for significant events like houses and weddings. This portfolio is liquid to the point of the distribution of the dividend and not tax-advantaged and can be purchased directly from the company through an agent such as www.directinvesting.com.

I also invest in my water company and electric company. Many companies provide a discount on equities for customers. This is good to take advantage of. Also, utility companies pay a healthy dividend.

One can start with a single share and purchase more in time when you have money or pass if you do not.

There are many categories.

- Defensive equities that serve to hold up during downturns
- Growth
- Large caps
- Mid caps
- Small caps
- Value
- Dividend plays
- International
- Speculative

Each has their place, but some require vigilance like the speculative equities, which can go from one hundred to one in months. And who wants to work harder or lose money.

The first concept is *dollar-cost averaging*. This is used with my non-Roth IRA, where I invest directly with the companies with little or no fees to buy. Dollar-cost averaging is the concept of buying a little at a time and buying more if the equity drops. Your basis is lowered and your yield gets better if it bears a dividend and it drops in value. Conversely, your shares appreciate if the stock goes up. You buy more at the low and less at the high.

Much of investing is patience. It is not emotional, so do not be emotional yourself but rather practice waiting because all equities rise and fall in a day, a week, or a month.

Many brokers allow alerts. Alerts are great if you see a good candidate to purchase or buy more, but it is near its fifty-two-week high. Set the alert where you would like to purchase.

If you hit the price, then buy. If not, you lose nothing. I do not buy as much as I can afford when it is rising. Rather, all equities will rise and fall for a variety of reasons. This is related to the concept of buy low and sell high.

Not all my accounts are precise. You buy near the low. I prefer to have a portion of this account in real estate investment trusts or REITs for short. REITs pay above average dividends. There are many types—office building owners, housing, and, my favorite, Plum Creek Timber. They own huge tracts of timber lands and also mineral and oil / gas rights.

Also, LTC, which is a REIT for assisted and senior care, is a good idea with the baby boomers getting older.

Add to your direct investments by the month by enrolling in a stock purchase plan direct from the company. I add to Coke, Procter & Gamble, and Well Fargo monthly.

Suggested for a fifty-year-old

Symbol	Quantity	Last Trade	Value within Asset	Percent of Allocation	Percent of Portfolio
Large Cap			$14,193.90	40.49%	
International			$3,400.83	9.70%	
Cash			$0.00	Get asset allocation recommendations 0.00%	
Mid/Small Cap			$13,628.67	38.87%	
Fixed Income			$745.22	2.13%	
Other			$3,090.36	8.81%	

15-Minute
Delayed Quotes

Humor Break
Marriage Counselor

A husband and wife came for counseling after twenty years of marriage. When asked what the problem was, the wife went into a passionate, painful tirade, listing every problem they had ever had in the twenty years they had been married.

She went on and on and on: neglect, lack of intimacy, emptiness, loneliness, feeling unloved and unlovable, an entire laundry list of unmet needs she had endured over the course of their marriage.

Finally, after allowing this to go on for a sufficient length of time, the therapist got up, walked around the desk and, after asking the wife to stand, embraced and kissed her passionately as her husband watched with a raised eyebrow. The woman shut up and quietly sat down as though in a daze.

The therapist turned to the husband and said, "This is what your wife needs at least three times a week. Can you do this?"

The husband thought for a moment and replied, "Well, I can drop her off here on Mondays and Wednesdays, but on Fridays, I fish."

INVESTING 301

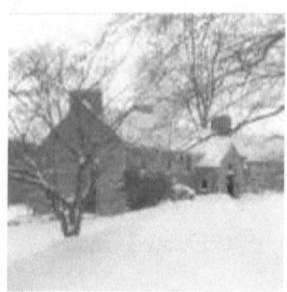

Trading Account

USE FILTERS TO screen for ideas. All brokerages have screening tools to use for free.

Do not fall in love with your investments. The most difficult concept is when to sell. I sometimes buy on bad news and often sell on good news.

Trading accounts are a way to stay liquid but also generate a little extra cash for small gains.

The next concept is market orders versus limit orders.

All equities will have a swing during a trading day. If you place a market order, you will buy high. I place an order below the bid using a limit order. I do this to take advantage of the intra-day swing. If the equity does not reach my low bid, I move on to another.

I like to trade for a specific goal like a new putter or a dinner with my wife. Stay hungry, my friends. What I look in an equity is the P/E (price-to-earnings ratio). That is its price divided by earnings. The P/E above twenty is not necessarily bad, because it is a trailing P/E. Look for the forward P/E. This could be a great opportunity if it is below twenty.

Do not try to "catch a falling knife." This can occur on an investment you own and want to dollar-cost average. If it falls, wait until the volume regulates to its normal level.

When dollar-cost averaging, one can place a trade that is good for sixty days. Place this trade at a significantly lower price than what you paid to open the investment.

A very important concept is the *stop loss*. This is intended to prevent losses due to unexpected changes in both the market and individual investments.

All short-term equities should be covered by a stop loss. I generally use a percentage of 7 to 10 percent of the asset less the price paid and enter a stop loss. This means that the unit will be sold automatically if it drops 7 to 10 percent.

Remember that all the research will not prevent losses. Some people get discouraged after taking a loss. Do not beat yourself up. I generally place them with securities that are short in focus and not intended for dollar-cost averaging.

Checklist for Buying an Equity

- The P/E is positive and under twenty.
- Not a maker of a single product (one-hit wonder).
- Pays a dividend (P/E divided by dividend yield is equal to two or below).
- Does not pay a dividend but has the possibility of substantial capital appreciation (must know that this is speculative in some cases).
- Geographic diversity (not dependent on a single country).
- Free cash flow is high.
- Management ownership in the company.
- Mutual funds have an investment in the company.
- Not near its fifty-two-week high.
- Not near its five-year high (room to grow).
- New products in research and development.
- Best in class.
- Management effectiveness.

If the overall economy is poor, use this time to buy bonds and add to an annuity or dollar cost up with high quality investments. Also, in tough times, reduce debt.

CDs (certificates of deposit) are very safe but pay better when the interest rates are higher. If the company does not pay a dividend, it should not be ruled out although it may not be a long-term hold.

I am not a day trader but rather a swing trader, which means I do not place a large trade hoping for appreciation in a short period of time. Instead, swing trades may not appreciate in a day, a month, or months, but over time, they appreciate for a healthy gain.

INVESTING 401

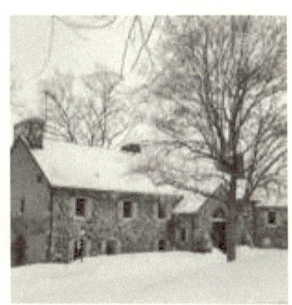

T HE FOURTH PART of my portfolio is a Roth IRA through ING Sharebuilder.com

To discover a candidate for a long-term dividend play divide the P/E by the dividend yield. If the result is two or below, it may be a good equity to begin a long-term investment.

There is another class of assets that I like. They are nondiversified, closed end funds. There are many dividend-paying, income-producing equities.

Two that are in my portfolio are managed by the Gabelli Group. Their symbols are GUT and GGN. The GUT invests in utilities and other assets, while GGN invests in gold and natural resources. They both pay an above average dividend monthly.

I have many monthly income funds from different broker/managers.

When looking at closed end funds for a dividend play, find out how long they have been paying the dividend. To be safe, I look for steady dividend payments for at least five years and preferably ten.

Recently, I began a program of buying top-notch American equities and selling profits into income producing equities. This has worked well for me. A few dollars reinvested dividends turn into real money over time.

ETFs (Exchange Traded Funds)

There are many different types investing in geography, types, etc. I hold positions in China, gas, gold and others. They are safer because you are buying a basket rather than a single entity but usually do not have a great dividend yield.

YOUR INVESTING 501

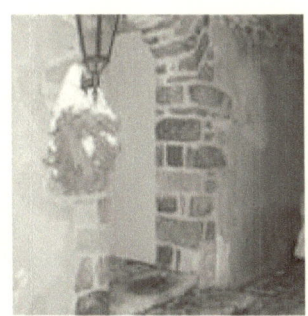

J OIN OR START an investment club with experienced traders. I learned the hard way to invest, and I was wrong in many cases. The worst thing that can happen is early success, where you feel invincible. My first trade was successful, and I thought that this was easy money.

Pride comes before a fall. Greed is a potent sin that will hurt you. Keep vigilant and learn.

Older people sometimes do not have the experience in executing trades but have the life experience to discern good from bad and job experiences in their fields, which give insight on a company or category. Try to join a very diversified group especially persons from abroad. They can give you information accrued from actually being in the country of origin.

To thoroughly investigate an opportunity, the club should read the current blogs. Much of this information can be tainted but read between the lines for some relevant ideas of what is going on with the subject.

We use the following to evaluate where a sponsor will do the homework and present it to the forum.

Stock/ETF Evaluation Form

- Name of company or ETF
- Symbol
- Industry
- Current price
- Fifty-two-week high
- Fifty-two-week low
- Five-year high
- Five-year low
- P/E
- Dividend yield
- EPS latest quarter
- Competitors
- Management ownership percent
- Mutual fund ownership percent
- Recent inside activity
- Why do you like this investment?

From this information, a group can discuss the investment. This data is the language of the private investor.

YOUR INVESTING 601

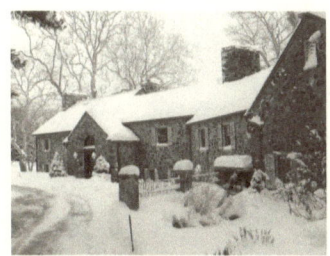

*S*ELF-DIRECTED IRA. USE a reputable broker to set this up for you. This type of IRA allows one to invest in real estate and precious metals: gold, silver, platinum, and palladium. Serious fines are levied if you misuse these or do not follow the rules.

YOUR CREDIT

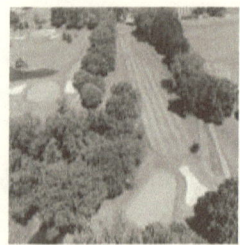

A N EXTREMELY IMPORTANT aspect of money management is *credit.* Insurance companies can rate your auto policy on your credit score. A bad credit score will haunt you and wipe away your gains. The inability to access credit will hurt your ability to purchase real property, which will be one of your bases to build wealth.

Companies will tease you into low interest lines of credit and slam you with fees if you are one day late in payment. Live within your means, and use credit within your ability to pay. There are situations to leverage, but debt can be good or bad.

I purchased two investment properties and renovated them using leverage. This is potentially good debt because the repayment was offset by depreciation of the properties.

Even though I was careful to make payments on time, I was hit with an increase because the company did not process the payment expeditiously. I eventually paid this off, but do not assume the company can wants to accept your payment on time. An important lesson—make the payment by mail a week ahead of time.

You can use credit to boost your credit and credit limit. This can be accomplished using two lines of credit. Remember to pay on time and fully. This is sort of like robbing Peter to pay Paul, but it can work if you are diligent.

Once you have established credit, do not close a line but get the balance down to zero. This tip came from a mortgage broker who works with credit scores and creditors every day.

The concept of good debt is debt that can subtract from taxes where home mortgage payments or depreciation on investment properties.

YOUR JOB

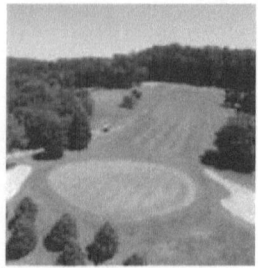

NO MATTER HOW humble a job is, it is a treasure. Of course, you are not going to like it every day, but it provides the fuel to build your pyramid of security.

Having a track record of work allows others to evaluate your willingness to accept responsibility. Again, it may seem trite and oversimplified, but in the words of Khalil Gibran, "Work is love made visible."

YOUR PARENTS

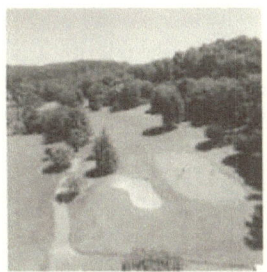

THERE MAY BE a need to buy a long-term care policy for a parent. This should be purchased before you have a crisis. It is less expensive if you do this early. Again, *time*.

My in-laws cared for my father-in-law after the passing of Barbara Schrey, my mother-in-law. He was doing well until felled by a stroke and she by cancer.

My sister-in-law, Susan Schrey, did a marvelous job of caring for him. They chose to keep him home although he showed symptoms of dementia.

Another friend, Barbara Bell, helped her parents move into assisted living. She is our dear friend who authored the following.

Caring for Your Parents
by Barbara Bell

The staggering statistic in America today is that 33 million people are caring for someone over 50 years of age. At only 43 years old, my mother had a debilitating stroke. It caused great pause in my life, and I wanted longingly, to re-capture those busy years while raising a child and working full time, to undo my selfishness. I would not recognize that my days with both of my parents would be shorter than I ever anticipated. The six years proceeding my mother's stroke, she would have another, we would move them from their home of 45 years. Time spent with them after these events would prove to be a blessing that would allow me the realization that the years behind me that I felt so guilty about would vanish quickly. The great memories of birthday parties and long hot summer days at the beach with them enabled me to remember that I DID include them in so much of my life while raising my son. In fact, these were some memories that they would cherish for their lifetime. When I was asked to inject a small portion of my experience within the confines of my dearest friend's first writings, I was honored. While I must admit, sitting down to write, I began to feel terror! What would I say? Where would I start? How would I end? A writer's most difficult questions. I asked Jim for a rubric, an outline, a minute sense of what he wanted to include. He is one of the most insightful men I know. He told me to explain that my weekly Sunday visits to my parents were invaluable. An easy trip for me to make a quick "checklist" of sorts to their needs, both physically and emotionally. It would also be a time for them to share an amazing account of the lives they lived together, so fully, for nearly 58 years! I encourage you to carve out a time, every week, preferably at the same time, on the same day, to just "visit." I mention the same day because looking back, I realized it was a time they too cherished and looked forward to every week. Although they lived independently, they lived in a place where on the weekends it became a bit desolate. From the maintenance man to the mailman, these warm souls would become a huge part of my father's life, as he talked to everyone. He also asked that I include the pain of my mother's very recent death. I still think that he asked me to include this, as in his brilliant brain, understanding the exercise would be a great healing process for me. Although he rarely credits himself for his caring ways, his underlying spirit is that of making sure that everyone else is taken care of. Mom's passing was pretty sudden. Although in the thick of it, a month's time felt like an eternity. She ended up in the care of a hospice. Hospice care could be a whole chapter in and of itself. This is where after almost 14 days with no food or water, her life would come to an end. The evening of her death, we knew that she was slipping away. My Dad, brothers, sister in law and Pastor would all be present. We would share an old hymn "It is well . . . with my soul." I would get up, move to her bedside, and gently lift her upper body, and kiss her on her head. This would be the place where she took her last breath. Later that night our beloved friend and Pastor would remind me, "This is not sad, my child, there is not another place she would have rather been than in the arms of her only daughter." It was as if it were yesterday. Grief was once looked upon as some voyage through different and discrete stages from denial to anger to depression and everything in between. The realization of loss, in the mind, gets re-played over and over. Generalizing death in terms of phases gives you a general picture, but even like death, it is unique in every person. I have sought the help of a professional, and for me the emotional support has been a blessing I could have never imagined. Emily Dickenson writes, "I measure every Grief I meet with narrow probing eyes—I wonder if it weighs like mine—or has an easier size." My 85-year-old Dad is who I concentrate on at this time. Wanting to rid his apartment of the wheelchair, he decided to donate it through our local pharmacy to and adult day care facility. What he didn't realize was that the journey through the narrow empty halls of their apartment with an empty wheelchair was almost more than he could bear. My heart was breaking when he told me this story, but the fact that he could express all this to me was a blessing and a gift. She was an amazing woman, a nurse, a wife, and a mother who always put everyone else first. She always "smiled through the pain." She often told me there is no problem too big to solve. Sometimes the answer comes more slowly than you wish, but the solution comes exactly when God wants it to. My advice, my friends, is as follows: Listen to your heart. Stay connected, do your homework, communicate, be patient and kind, and always remember they were there for you, when no one else would be. The bond is one that will remain unbroken, and even if the relationship is not one that you feel is perfect, work on it, ask questions, let them tell you stories of their past as these moments are windows into the eyes of their souls. I write this as I prepare to go to the funeral home and pick up my mother's ashes. None of us could seem to muster up the courage to take this final step. It is a process, one where "taking baby steps" feel much like climbing the tallest mountain. Take them slowly and deliberately and somehow you will come through the other side.

"For what is it to die but to stand naked in the wind and melt into the sun? And what is it to cease breathing, but to free the breath from its restless tides, that it may rise and expand and seek God unencumbered? Only when you drink from the river of silence shall you indeed sing, and when you reach the mountain top, then shall you begin to climb. And when the earth shall claim your limbs, then shall you truly dance"

YOUR FINANCIAL SECURITY

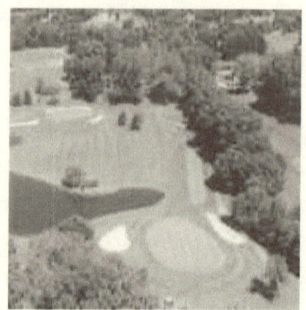

A MUST IS BOTH a short-term and a *long-term* disability policy. If your company does not provide these, purchase one early on the open market. I was fortunate to have a policy in place when MS hit me. It eases the impact of illness or accidents

YOUR REAL PROPERTY

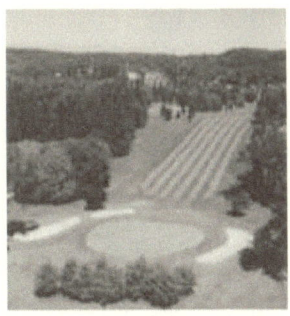

YOUR HOME IS not a piggy bank. It is an essential builder of wealth.

Be careful to use your equity. Watch home equity loans. A default will cause a foreclosure just the same as a primary.

I have two investment properties that I purchased from HUD with the help of my brother-in-law, the brilliant Guy Matteo. Guy took a turn as president of Pennsylvania's Association of Realtors. They were foreclosed and in terrible condition

I used two groups of contractors simultaneously.

In retrospect, I should have listened to Guy and gotten three written quotes for each milestone.

They were completed and tenanted after much anxiety.

Try to be cash positive.

Depreciation is a huge tax benefit.

Keep accurate records of what you put into them and save receipts.

YOUR DRIVING SKILLS

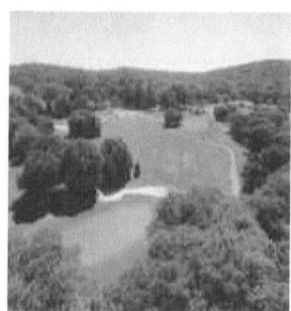

*Y*OUR DRIVING SKILLS are important for your health and wallet. I learned to drive working a taxicab. Very simple—get from point A to point B without causing damage to yourself or others.

Bob works hard at the plant and spends two nights each week bowling and plays golf every Saturday.

His wife thinks he's pushing himself too hard, so for his birthday, she takes him to a local strip club.

The doorman at the club greets them and says, "Hey, Bob! How ya doin'?"

His wife is puzzled and asks if he's been to this club before.

"Oh no," says Bob. "He's in my bowling team."

When they are seated, a waitress asks Bob if he'd like his usual and brings over a Budweiser. His wife is becoming increasingly uncomfortable and says, "How did she know that you drink Budweiser?"

"I recognize her. She's the waitress from the golf club. I always have a Bud at the end of the first nine, honey."

A stripper then comes over to their table, throws her arms around Bob, starts to rub herself all over him, and says, "Hi, Bobby. Want your usual table dance, big boy?"

Bob's wife, now furious, grabs her purse and storms out of the club. Bob follows and spots her getting into a cab. Before she can slam the door, he jumps in beside her. Bob tries desperately to explain how the stripper must have mistaken him for someone else, but his wife is having none of it. She is screaming at him at the top of her lungs, calling him every four-letter word in the book.

The cabby turns around and says, "Geez, Bob, you picked up a real b—tch this time."

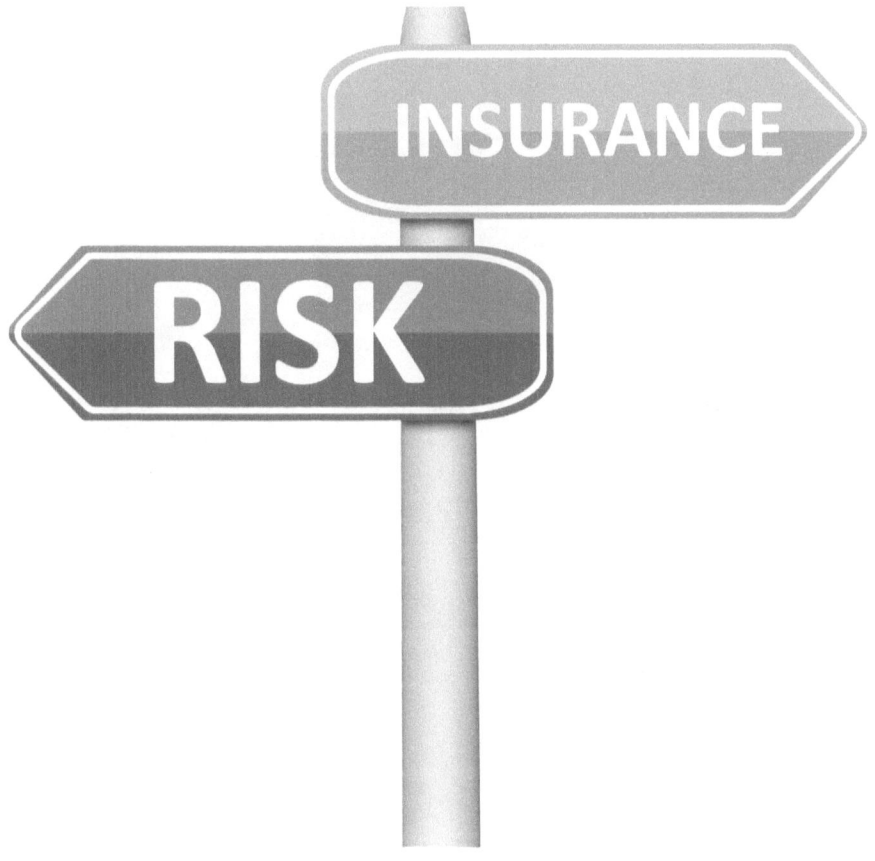

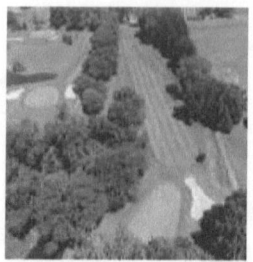

L IFE INSURANCE EQUALS to your mortgage.
Liability insurance on your cars equals to your wealth.

Short—and Long-Term Disability Policy:

Long-term care policy starting at age 45 and/or a policy for parents

YOUR SIGNIFICANT OTHER

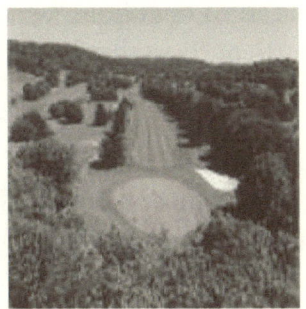

A HUSBAND TAKES HIS wife to play her first game of golf. Of course, the wife promptly whacked her first shot right through the window of the biggest house adjacent to the course.

The husband cringed. "I warned you to be careful! Now we'll have to go up there, find the owner, apologize, and see how much your lousy drive is going to cost us."

So the couple walked up to the house and knocked on the door. A warm voice said, "Come on in."

When they opened the door, they saw the damage that was done: glass was all over the place, and a broken antique bottle was lying on its side near the broken window.

A man reclining on the couch asked, "Are you the people that broke my window?"

"Uh . . . yeah, sir. We're sure sorry about that," the husband replied.

"Oh, no apology is necessary. Actually I want to thank you . . .

You see, I'm a genie, and I've been trapped in that bottle for a thousand years. Now that you've released me, I'm allowed to grant three wishes. I'll give you each one wish, but if you don't mind, I'll keep the last one for myself."

"Wow, that's great!" the husband said. He pondered a moment and blurted out, "I'd like a million dollars a year for the rest of my life."

"No problem," said the genie. "You've got it. It's the least I can do. And I'll guarantee you a long, healthy life! And now you, young lady, what do you want?" the genie asked.

"I'd like to own a gorgeous home complete with servants in every country in the world," she said.

"Consider it done," the genie said. "And your homes will always be safe from fire, burglary, and natural disasters!"

"And now," the couple asked in unison, "what's your wish, genie?"

"Well, since I've been trapped in that bottle and haven't been with a woman in more than a thousand years, my wish is to have sex with your wife."

The husband looked at his wife and said, "Gee, honey, you know we both now have a fortune and all those houses . . . What do you think?"

She mulled it over for a few moments and said, "You know, you're right.

Considering our good fortune, I guess I wouldn't mind, but what about you, honey?"

"You know I love you, sweetheart," said the husband. "I'd do the same for you!"

So the genie and the woman went upstairs, where they spent the rest of the afternoon enjoying each other in every way. After about three hours of nonstop sex, the genie rolled over and looked directly into her eyes and asked, "How old are you and your husband?"

"Why, we're both thirty-five," she responded breathlessly.

"NO SH—T," he said. "Thirty-five years old and both of you still believe in genies?"

Your significant others must be remembered. They may have different values and risk aversion. Communicate on a regular basis. Dedicate time without distractions

Humor Break

Every wife is a "mistress" for her husband—
"miss" for one hour and "stress" for the rest twenty-three hours!

There are two times when a man doesn't understand a woman— before marriage and after marriage.

My husband and I divorced over religious differences.
He thought he was God, and I didn't.

Husband throwing darts at his wife's photo and not even a single one hitting the target . . .
From another room, Wife called the husband, "Honey, what are you doing?"
Husband said, "Missing you!"

Thought for the Day
Women are like phones:
They like to be held, talked to, and touched often.
But push the wrong button and you're disconnected.

Difference between Complete and Finish
People say there is no difference between *complete* and *finish*. But there is.
When you marry the right one, you are *complete*.
And when you marry the wrong one, you are *finished*.
And when the right one catches you with the wrong one, you are . . . *completely finished!*

Romantic SMS
She sends the following message:
My love if you're sleeping, send me your dreams.
If you're smiling, send me your smile.
If you're crying, send me your tears.
I love you.

He replied, "I'm in the toilet. What do I send?"
- - - - - - - - - -

There are three kinds of men in the world:
Some remain single and make wonders happen,
Some have girlfriends and see wonders happen,
The rest get married and wonder what happened!

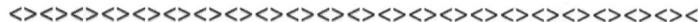

The ABC

After being married for thirty years, a wife asked her husband to describe her.

He looked at her slowly then said, "You're A, B, C, D, E, F, G, H . . . I, J, K."

She asks, "What does that mean?"

He said, "Adorable, beautiful, cute, delightful, elegant, fancy, gorgeous honey.

She smiled happily and said, "Oh, that's so lovely . . . What about I, J, K?"

He said, "I'm just kidding!"

His eye is still swollen, but it will get better.

*   *   *

At the cocktail party, one woman said to another, "Aren't you wearing your wedding ring on the wrong finger?"

The other replied, "Yes, I am. I married the wrong man."

Summation

Buy equities and ETFs of companies that you understand.

Do not chase stocks but rather buy a little and average up.

Set alerts.

There is room for speculation, and inexpensive stocks can go off the board.

Equities have no memory.

Watch the world around you.

Buy bonds as you get older.

Take care of your health.

Visit a dentist.

Drive slower.

Best of luck.

Final Humor Break

Irish Discretion

Six retired Irishmen are playing poker in O'Leary's apartment, when Paddy Murphy loses five hundred pounds on a single hand, clutches his chest, and drops dead at the table.

Showing respect for their fallen brother, the other five continue playing, standing up.

Michael O'Conner looks around and asks, "Oh, me boys, someone got to tell Paddy's wife. Who will it be?"

They draw cards for the task. Paul Gallagher picks the two of clubs and becomes the one to tell Mrs. Murphy the bad news. They tell him to be discreet, be gentle, don't make a bad situation any worse.

"Discreet? I'm the most discreet Irishman you'll ever meet. Discretion is me middle name. Leave it to me."

Gallagher goes over to Murphy's house and knocks on the door. Mrs. Murphy answers and asks what he wants.

Gallagher declares, "Your husband just lost five hundred pounds and is afraid to come home."

"Tell him to drop dead!" says Murphy's wife.

"I'll go tell him," says Gallagher.

APPENDIX A

Template for an Investment Club

HaverBroomTown Investment Club Proposal

THE PURPOSE IN addition to building wealth is to inform young people how to manage their accounts for retirement and financial needs throughout their lives.

The parties agree that a price of the private placement of shares will have a value of twenty-five dollars, with three dollars collected monthly to cover fees accrued in the purchasing of equities for the purpose of capital appreciation of shares and the reinvestment of all capital gains and dividends.

The parties agree that there should be meetings held bimonthly on the fifteenth of the month, where a reporting of activity will occur and discussions can be held on new investments, the selling of equities to take profit/loss, or other business and that the equities will be held by a discount broker such as E-Trade, which allows clubs to operate.

All participants will have daily access unless an early divestment occurs, and the password will be changed and the remaining participants will be e-mailed the new one.

The parties agree that the first placement will begin and end in a three-year period.

The relationship will be joint tenancy with rights of survivorship.

For tax purposes, each individual is responsible for their own taxes according to the number of shares owned.

Parties can purchase additional shares at the twenty-eight dollars before and during the initial series.

During the next series, additional shares can be purchased at the twenty-eight-dollar level for owners of record during the primary series, but new investor's price will be at the new basis or twenty-eight dollars, whichever is higher.

A party can decide to not participate for shares but no longer than three consecutive months. If no investment is found for three consecutive months, the participant can buy back in for twenty-five-dollar penalty to avoid early divestments.

For vesting purposes, early divestment is discouraged. You do not accrue share equity if you do not participate that month, and early divestment returns your principal to date of your shares minus ninety-nine dollars the first year, sixty-six dollars during the second year, and thirty-three dollars during the third year, and all dividends accrued.

Shares divested because of hardship or other reasons can be purchased by other participants for twenty-five dollars free of the three-dollar fee by payment to the individual directly with a required email to the treasurer.

The price of the shares will be realized after the initial three years by dividing the total equity by the total number of shares.

The decision to begin a new cycle is then voted on where each vote is dependent on your total shares creating a new basis. The original fee will remain the same plus the three-dollar fee for existing members and the new basis for new members that begin the second iteration plus the three dollars, whichever is greater.

Divestment after the first three-year period will be paid on the completed new-share basis free of penalties for member of good standing if they decide to not participate in the subsequent series.

Payments can be made by check or PayPal.

My personal check list is this:

Checklist for Buying an Equity

- The P/E is positive and under twenty.
- Not a maker of a single product (one-hit wonder).
- Pays a dividend (P/E divided by dividend yield is equal to two or below).
- Does not pay a dividend but has the possibility of substantial capital appreciation (must know that this is speculative in some cases).
- Geographic diversity (not dependent on a single country).
- Free cash flow is high.
- Management ownership in the company.
- Mutual funds have an investment in the company.
- Not near its fifty-two-week high.
- Not near its five-year high (room to grow).
- New products in research and development.
- Best in class.

- Management effectiveness.
- Market is rising.
- A portion of the account S/B in gold and gold miners to hedge against inflation and/or the drop in the US dollar.

The purchasing of equities will be voted on by the members after consideration of what type of investment it is.

- Speculative buy
- Long-term buy
- Watch list
- Purchase
- Sell
- Purchase with intent to dollar-cost average
- Dividend play

In order to vote on stock purchases, a stock eval form S/B filled out or sent to all thru the distribution.

The quantity for purchases will also be voted on and executed during the last two weeks of the month, depending on the type, ex-dividend date, and other criteria to get the lowest price for the purchase.

Along with the purchase, the sell price will also be established and a stop loss established to protect the investment.

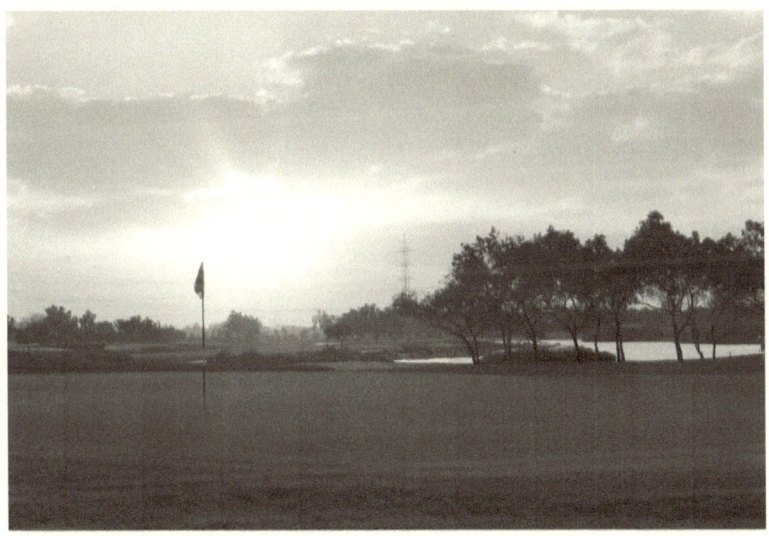

INDEX

JAMES WILLIAM SCHWARZ

P

Philadelphia Inquirer, 22
Plum Creek Timber, 34
portfolio, 15-16, 31, 33, 39
pound-cost averaging, 14
price-to-earnings ratio (P/E), 36-37, 39, 62
pride, 41
profit, 39, 61

R

real estate, 15, 34, 43
Reid, Andy, 22
Riegel, Robert Henry "Skee," 20
risk, 14-15, 31, 56

S

Schrey, Barbara, 47
Schrey, Susan, 47
shares, 14, 34, 61-62
Smiley, Frank, 19
stocks, 15, 31, 34, 59, 63
stop loss, 37, 63
swing trade, 38

T

teeth, 26

V

Vanderslice, Ted, 28
Vanderslice, Terry, 23
Vanguard, 30, 32
volatility, 31